NOT YOUR AVERAGE RUNNER™

NOT YOUR AVERAGE RUNNER™

WHY YOU'RE NOT TOO FAT TO RUN, AND THE SKINNY ON HOW TO START TODAY

JILL ANGIE

NEW YORK

LONDON • NASHVILLE • MELBOURNE • VANCOUVER

NOT YOUR AVERAGE RUNNER™

Why You're Not Too Fat to Run and the Skinny on How to Start Today

Published in New York, New York, by Morgan James Publishing in partnership with Difference Press. Morgan James is a trademark of Morgan James, LLC. www.MorganJamesPublishing.com

The Morgan James Speakers Group can bring authors to your live event. For more information or to book an event visit The Morgan James Speakers Group at www.TheMorganJamesSpeakersGroup.com.

ISBN 9781683504603 paperback
ISBN 9781683504610 eBook
Library of Congress Control Number: 2017902310

Cover and Interior Design by:
Chris Treccani
www.3dogcreative.net

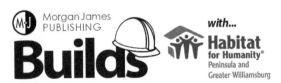

In an effort to support local communities, raise awareness and funds, Morgan James Publishing donates a percentage of all book sales for the life of each book to Habitat for Humanity Peninsula and Greater Williamsburg.

Get involved today! Visit
www.MorganJamesBuilds.com

This book is dedicated to all my family and friends, for believing in my wildest dreams and helping me bring them to life.

Thank you.

TABLE OF CONTENTS

ABOUT THIS BOOK

"Run when you can, walk if you have to, crawl if you must; just never give up."
DEAN KARNAZES

I f you're reading this book, I assume you either want to learn more about running or you accidentally clicked the "Buy now" button on your Kindle and you're silently cursing your itchy trigger finger. Regardless of the reason, here we are and I think we've got a lot to discuss.

First of all, what is this book about? On the surface, it's about running. Specifically, how a woman carrying a few (or many) extra pounds can successfully become a runner in the body she has, right now. But this is also a book about side effects. Running is addictive, and after you've been doing it for a while, people will begin to notice undeniable changes in your behavior. They might not say anything to your face, but behind your back they'll be talking:

"She just seems so much more confident lately–do you think she's had work done?"

"Perhaps it's a new pair of heels? Lately she just seems … taller."

"Maybe she's having an affair. Three times a week, she disappears at lunch and comes back looking so satisfied. And a little sweaty."

Confidence: a classic side-effect of a running addiction.

But I digress. First, we need to chat about obesity, self-esteem, and Instagram. Trust me–they are related.

It's no secret that waistlines are growing. Walk down any street and you'll see plenty of people who meet the medical definition of obese. This phenomenon isn't limited to the US–the world is growing larger, and the trend doesn't appear to be slowing. Experts point to numerous causes: poor diets that rely too much on convenience (usually processed) foods, enormous portions, sprawling suburbs set up for driving instead of walking, and even the diet industry itself. And they're right–these issues are all part of the problem, along with dozens more that I haven't named.

But there is another fundamental contributor, something that most people overlook when trying to understand why we are busting out of our clothes, airplane seats and restaurant chairs: self-esteem, or rather, the lack of it among women and girls in this country.

You could argue that low self-esteem is a symptom of the obesity epidemic, rather than the cause. I agree, to a point, but it's more like the chicken and the egg–which came first? We'll probably never know, and it doesn't really matter. Low self-esteem and obesity are inextricably linked in our society.

Judging and shaming others for their physical imperfections has become a national pastime. Don't believe me? Pick up any tabloid and you're guaranteed to see photos of a Hollywood star who has dared to publicly frolic in a bikini, brazenly exposing two square inches of cellulite on an otherwise perfect butt. This phenomenon isn't limited to those in the public eye. A quick look at Instagram or Facebook will almost certainly yield snapshots of overweight and/or oddly dressed people, accompanied by a snidely worded status update mocking them. Why? If you're feeling fat, ugly, or in any way *less than perfect* yourself, it's easy to look at someone else's body or sense of style and think "I may have flaws, but at least I don't look like *that*."

But as cruel as women can be when judging others, we never criticize anyone more harshly than ourselves. If your girlfriend gains five pounds, you console her with something like "Don't worry, it's only water weight." But if you do the same? The little voice inside your head is more likely to sound something like "You lazy piece of crap, you're a complete failure at life." If you think I'm exaggerating, eavesdrop on your internal dialogue sometime. I mean *really* listen. You'll be shocked at what you say to yourself. If your best friend spoke to you that way, your friendship wouldn't last long–so why is it OK to treat yourself so poorly?

We're constantly told that being overweight is a character flaw, and we believe it. We claim it as truth, as factual as the color of our eyes or the size of our feet. The earth is round. Being fat makes you a terrible person.

Obsession with perfection is everywhere: magazines, TV, internet, billboards, social media. The messages are insidious, and before we realize what's happened, the thought "You don't measure up" becomes an unshakable truth. We understand that the flawless images we see everywhere are a result of good lighting and Photoshop, but those nasty, whispery voices in our heads have already bought into the dogma of perfection with gusto, and they are not afraid to speak up and make their opinions heard.

So we spend hours and hours scrolling through Instagram or Facebook, painstakingly searching for inspiration and advice to help us come closer to the standard of perfection.

Posting photos of extremely fit women as fitness inspiration (or as the practice is commonly known, fitspiration) seems like an innocuous, perhaps even useful, pastime. What's wrong with looking at someone else's success and using it to inspire your own? Nothing, if that's what's truly taking place, but most of the time, it means comparing our own everyday bodies and lives to someone else's (Photoshopped) highlight reels, and then finding our own situation lacking.

One of my particular favorites is the catchphrase "Strong is the new skinny" that's currently sweeping the internet. Taken at face value, this seems like a great motivational truism. No longer do we need to be skinny to be accepted in society! Be strong! Kick butt! Take no prisoners!

Except … every time I've seen this slogan, it is plastered over a picture of an impossibly fit model with unreasonably low body fat. Don't get me wrong–the dedication and effort that it takes to achieve and maintain that type of body is admirable. It's just unrealistic for the vast majority of women (i.e., women whose job description is not "fitness model"). Strong really is the new skinny, because the new standard is just as (or perhaps even more) unattainable as the old. In addition to being impossibly thin, we now need to have rippling muscles and the ability to do a one-handed pushup while rocking a bikini. We're not just fat anymore–we're fat, weak, and uncoordinated. Why even bother? Pass the cupcakes, please.

When we believe we're not worthy, we stop treating ourselves with respect, which includes good nutrition, kind self-talk, regular exercise, and so on. Yes, obesity may be a result of overeating, but why is everyone eating so much in the first place? There's certainly no lack of information about proper nutrition and portion sizes available to the general population. But in the absence of feeling good about ourselves, external mood enhancers such as food, alcohol, or shopping (to name a few) are a quick fix. Food is particularly easy to abuse in this way, because it's inexpensive, widely available, and socially acceptable. Bad day at work? All it takes is a few quarters in the vending machine to get temporary relief. Unfortunately, the reprieve is short-lived. Shortly after the snack wrappers are in the trash, guilt settles in for a nice long visit. And therein lies our chicken-or-egg dilemma–self-medicating with too much food results in the very thing that triggered the low self-esteem in the first place.

What's a girl to do? A strict diet and exercise plan might take the pounds off, but if your deepest beliefs about yourself are unchanged, it won't be long before you'll find yourself partying with your buddies Ben & Jerry late at night. True change comes from within. Instead of searching outwardly for a reflection of what makes you a person of value–your size, appearance, clothes, or the balance in your bank account–you must start believing you are perfect and lovable merely because you exist. That no matter what anyone else thinks, you matter. You are beautiful, fabulous and amazing exactly as you are this very moment.

Of course, that's easier said than done. How can I just change my mind? I've been practicing all of those mean thoughts about myself for years! I'm so good at thinking that way!

This is where running enters the picture. Once upon a time, I was exactly where you are. Running changed all of that, but it didn't happen overnight. I'm hoping that my experiences will help speed up the process for you.

I've been a runner, off and on, for 20 years. I started in the summer of 1998, running laps around my block. At the time, I tipped the scales at 200 pounds, give or take (mostly give), and my block was roughly a half mile around, at least according to the odometer on my '97 Saturn. This was before the era of smart phones and GPS watches, a time when heart rate monitors were just becoming mainstream, and well before cute workout clothes came in anything larger than a size L. I'd never even seen anyone my size running in public! So I ran in too-tight leggings, stretched so thin you could almost see my leg tattoo, and covered up my body in men's cotton t-shirts that I picked up for $3 apiece at the local outlet store–shirts so enormous they hung almost to my knees. A cheap digital watch timed my intervals, and more than once I almost fell flat on my face because I was too busy counting down the last five seconds to watch where I was going.

I was slow and couldn't run continuously for more than thirty seconds at a time for those first few weeks. It was difficult and uncomfortable, and most of the time I thought I was going to pass out. More than one person told me I would destroy my knees by running. (Side note: most of the people that describe all the terrible things that will happen to you if you run are not actually runners, which makes them unqualified to give you advice. You should ignore them). I worried that my leggings would eventually just split right down the center seam as I catapulted myself across a big puddle, and I wondered if I would ever be able to run more than a minute without stopping to walk. Once, I was chased by a dog and another time was heckled by two little kids that thought the sight of me chugging down the sidewalk was the funniest thing they'd ever seen. And on one memorable evening, I stepped out in front of a minivan moments before the driver made an unexpected right turn. She saw me just in time to hit the brakes, but not quickly enough to avoid sending me sprawling on the pavement. Fortunately for both of us, I didn't sustain any serious bodily injuries. My faithful yellow Sony Sports Discman, however, was another story.

I could have used any of these events as excuses not to run, but I felt so powerful when I ran those first laps around the block. Thirty-second intervals turned into 60-second intervals, and pretty soon I was able to run one lap without stopping. I didn't lose a lot of weight through this process–maybe five to ten pounds–but I slowly worked up to running a little more each time. Every milestone reached built up my self-esteem a teeny bit more. I began to tell people I was a runner. It felt incredible.

After a few weeks, I was able to do an entire lap of the block without walking, then two. That fall, I entered a 5K, crossing the finish line in about forty-two minutes. I was nearly dead last and it felt like the sweetest victory of my life. Especially when my best friend's seven-year-old son joined me a few steps before the finish line and crossed with me, his arms waving in the air like we'd just finished a marathon. My self-confidence was at an all-time high. It was a magical experience–and I wanted to hold onto that feeling forever.

The next day, I rested. Then one more day, for good measure. On day three, I'd love to say I laced up my shoes and hit the streets, but I just … didn't. In fact, I didn't run again for a few years. I have no real explanation for why I just stopped doing something that gave me so much joy, other than the mean girl in my head wanted to feel good by eating pizza and ice cream *right this second*, rather than go to all the effort of overcoming the gravity of the couch, changing into unflattering workout clothes, and sweating it out for at least fifteen minutes before the feel-good endorphins kicked in. She also has a lot of opinions, most of which are in the "you'll never be a real runner so why even bother" genre. She's kind of a jerk that way.

(Spoiler alert: my inner mean girl is named Whinona. You'll meet her later.)

Fast forward to 2001 and I began commuting a hundred and twenty-five miles, round trip, each day to a desk job. I'm sure you can do the math–an extra two to three hours per day behind the wheel of my car did nothing but increase the size of my butt. Remembering my short-lived glory days as a runner, I joined a gym near my office, and began to run some half-hearted intervals on the treadmill after work. A year later, I sold my house and moved five miles from my employer, to an apartment next to a beautiful bike path along the Schuylkill River. Running was back in my life, and the old magic began to return. I met my future husband, a long-distance runner and triathlete. Jackpot! We hit the trail together every weekend, and after several months, I was able to run a few miles without stopping. The day I managed to run seven miles in a row, I felt like a complete rock star. Nothing was going to stop me this time around!

Buoyed by my success, I signed up to do the 2004 Broad Street Run, a popular local race that stretches ten miles down the very center of Philadelphia. With the race about six months out, and considering that I was already running seventy percent of the distance, it seemed there was plenty of time to train. I set a goal of finishing in two hours or less ... and stopped running again.

It wasn't pretty, but I did cross the finish line, and that was my last run for a few years. Inevitably, I began again. Got hooked again. Stopped again. Lather, rinse, repeat.

Fast forward to present day, and I run consistently at least three times a week. Although I'm a bit faster and sleeker than 1998, I'm still a chunky back-of-the-packer, and proud of it! While it is likely that I'll never win any races (unless I'm still running when I'm 70–the field is much smaller at that age), I *always* finish.

You might wonder why I'm qualified to give advice about running, self-esteem, or anything even remotely related to those topics. After two decades and hundreds of miles I know a thing or two about both. I also know how to pick myself up, dust myself off and start again. I've been exactly where you are now, and have come through it.

The most important lesson I've learned over the years is that running is a metaphor for success. Take things one step at a time, keep moving forward (even if you have to walk or crawl), and eventually you'll reach your goal. Let go of unrealistic expectations while simultaneously pushing yourself out of your comfort zone. That's the magic formula.

When you think about your workouts this way, the thrill of possibility lies just beyond the next step, even when it sucks. Even in the rain, the snow, or the crushing heat and humidity that passes for summer in Southeastern Pennsylvania. It's all good. It's better than good. It is a high like no other.

It's that moment when you realize you are so freaking *strong* and who cares about being skinny. When you stop obsessing about whether your butt cheeks are shaking with each step and realize that those glorious glutes are what power you forward. When you have to double check that your feet are actually touching the ground with each step, because for a moment there it seemed like you might actually be flying. When you find yourself unapologetically weeping at the end of a long run, in awe of your own strength, courage and endurance.

Yeah, that feeling. You can't get that from a cupcake (I've tried).

It doesn't matter how many times you start over, as long as you do. Running will always be there for you, and with it, your self-assurance. You can always begin again. It is never, ever too late. To quote John Bingham, "The miracle isn't that I finished. The miracle is that I had the courage to start."

So be brave, lace up those shoes, and let's get down to business. It's time to run your way back to self-esteem, confidence, and fabulosity.

But first, download and print the Not Your Average Runner Manifesto, and hang it on your bathroom mirror, on the fridge, on the dashboard of your car, or on the back of the front door - for a little extra support when you need it.

www.NotYourAverageRunner.com/Manifesto

RUNNERS RUN

How do you know you've become a runner? When you realize you own more sneakers than any other type of shoe. When you find yourself discussing the pros and cons of various refueling gels with a straight face. When paying more for compression tights than a designer handbag seems completely normal. I could go on, but the best answer is this:

If you run, you are a runner.

That's it. Fast or slow, short distances or long, twice a month or twice a day, runners run. Whether for thirty miles or thirty seconds, they just run. Regardless of your fitness level, body shape, or weight, you become a runner as soon as you put on your shoes, step out the front door, and run. Voila, you're in the club.

FINDING YOUR BLISS

Everyone that exercises has a reason for pursuing the particular type of workout that appeals to them. For swimmers, it might be the relaxing feel of the water against their skin. For indoor cyclists, the loud music and group atmosphere is energizing. Golfers enjoy the time in nature, or the challenge of competing against themselves. Bullfighters? Well, I'm not really sure why. It all sounds a little crazy to me, but they must get something out of it.

Truly understanding why I choose to run has made it much easier to get out the door on days when I'm busy, tired, or would rather binge-watch TV on Netflix. When I first started, it was strictly an efficient mode of burning calories. Then I realized how great I felt after a run, both physically and mentally, and I started chasing that feeling. Over the years, running has brought a mountain of self-confidence into my life, along with the sweet relief of no longer worrying what anyone else thinks about me. Trust me—once you are free from the burden of others' opinions, the world is your oyster. And the more I run, the more liberated I become.

But mostly, I've realized that I truly love everything about running. And I mean everything: even when it hurts, when the rain is pouring down, or the heat and humidity are so intense that I break a sweat just tying my shoes, I still love it. It's all part of the experience. It is my bliss.

Dictionary.com defines bliss as "supreme happiness; utter joy or contentment," and that pretty much sums up it how it feels to me. That doesn't mean I never get injured, or feel fatigue and frustration. Far from it. Sometimes my body gets so tired I'm not sure how I'm going to take another step (that's when I picture myself as Rocky, running through the streets of South Philly with kids cheering me on. Works like a charm every time).

Bliss co-exists with all of the discomfort and somehow makes it easy to bear. Bliss rocks.

At this point, you're probably rolling your eyes, thinking "Yeah, that's fine for you, but I don't feel bliss – or anything even remotely close–when I run. All I feel is sweaty, tired and frankly, a little pissed off."

Fair enough. I expected some resistance, so I called on my running friends from around the country, women of all shapes, sizes, lifestyles and fitness levels, to share the reasons they run:

> "My favorite part about running is those moments, and they do happen, when you are in such a rhythm that it seems the world is moving by you

instead of you running through it. It's an amazing feeling. I love being in the groove of running. I love how it benefits my physical and emotional health. I love the opportunity it gives me to be in nature just thinking, processing and pondering without interruption. I love the conversations you can have with a good running buddy. I love being reminded that I *can* do *anything*."

McKenzie D., Bend, OR

"Once I started running consistently, I fell in love with it. There IS such a thing as a runner's high. Not only do you feel a great sense of accomplishment after finishing a run or reaching a new goal, but there is also something that happens chemically inside me when I run consistently. Sometimes, I just want to drop what I am doing and run...even when I am nicely dressed and on my way into work, my body says *run*. Having a spontaneous urge to do something healthy is such a great feeling."

- Abby S., Westchester, PA

"It means I've accomplished a personal goal. It means that I get to be proud of myself. And it means that I get to face the voice inside that tells me to take it easy and tell it to be quiet while I put on my shoes, head out the door, and go move my body. The resulting sense of pride and accomplishment is why I do it."

– GINA D., SANTA ROSA, CA

"Running does make me feel happier and more fit, which helps me feel better about myself and more confident. Again, since we're being honest here, when I feel confident I'm more likely to seduce my husband, take risks at work, speak in public … it's a good cycle."

– AMANDA R., WAYNE, PA

Each of these women has found her own personal running nirvana–she knows exactly what she's getting from the experience and it's more than just burning calories or losing weight. It's confidence, and it keeps her coming back again and again.

My advice to you is to really understand why you run, or why you *want* to run. Make a list, and keep adding to it over time. Review it on those days when you think there are too many other things you'd rather do than run, or when it seems like the world is conspiring against you. It's OK if you don't know all the answers right now, all you need to do is give it some thought.

Some days it will be tough to find your happy place while running, especially in the beginning. This is to be expected. Even if you know exactly why you're out there pounding the pavement, the future payoff might not feel worth the effort of the present moment. Keep going anyway, and focus on what *is* going well. It might be the simple fact that you got your butt out the door at 6am when you wanted to sleep for another half-hour, or that your shins don't hurt quite as much as last time. Whatever it is, find it, grab it, and celebrate it.

Just do me a favor–don't ever use running as a reason to beat yourself up for being inadequate. If your workout just didn't go as planned, focusing on what *did* go well is a heck of a lot less painful than being pissed off because you didn't set a personal record. You can deconstruct why things went south, and use that information to learn and improve, but please don't use it as evidence of failure. There is no such thing as a bad run, only the one you didn't do.

TAKING THE FIRST STEP

Martin Luther King, Jr. once said "You don't have to see the whole staircase. Just take the first step."

Wise words.

But even taking that first step can be daunting, particularly if you're brand new to the sport. The human mind can be quite contradictory: wanting to try something that we believe will be rewarding, while simultaneously reminding us that we're likely to fail, so why even bother?

Many women believe they are not well-suited to running, based on the simple fact that when they do, they can't run very far. Often this is just due to a lack of conditioning, or trying to go too fast, too soon. Running is hard work, and it takes awhile for your body–especially your heart, lungs, and legs–to adapt to the challenge. Just because you can't run for 20 minutes your first time out doesn't mean you're not meant to be a runner, it just means you've got work to do.

Consistency is critical to improvement, and one of the easiest ways to ensure that you're keeping up with your workouts is to follow a training schedule. For example, if your goal is to run three miles, you might choose a training plan with three runs per week, each week gradually increasing time, distance, and/or speed until you achieve your goal. But looking at your desired end state vs. your current fitness level can be a bit overwhelming. And what do most of us do when faced with a seemingly insurmountable challenge? Panic, hit the snooze button, and vow to start tomorrow. Repeat for two months. Chastise yourself when you realize you are no closer to your goal.

I've got a better idea: just envision the very first step of the staircase. Instead of freaking out about how far you are from your goal, concern yourself with what you need to do today, or even the next ten minutes. That might be as simple as putting your shoes on and going outside, or driving to the gym. Then worry about the next step. Gina D. sums it up perfectly:

"What I love more than anything else about running is the lesson it teaches me to take life in small steps and to focus on the moment. I liken the experience to knitting. You can only knit a project one stitch at a time, so you better learn to enjoy each stitch, otherwise you'll get to the end of the project and will have hated doing it the entire time. When I run and look way ahead at how far I have to go, it can become overwhelming, so I focus on just one step in front of me and stop looking at the overall distance. It takes me further that way."

A friend once asked me if I could see improvement in my performance from week to week. I thought about it for a moment, and answered "No." Unless you are an absolute beginner, a week is really too short of time to see measurable changes. But if I look back at where I was three months, six months or two years ago, the improvement is immediately visible. It feels great to see that difference, and realize how far I've come. If I'd spent every week of the past two years looking for evidence of change, however, I would have been sorely disappointed. Placing too much importance on seeing progression can be a huge de-motivator. Just ask any woman who has been desperately trying to lose weight, only to see a big goose-egg on the scale week after week–if her only reason for making healthy choices every day is to see the number on the scale decrease, you can bet she'll be face-down in a pan of lasagna before too long. The same goes for running. If your final result is more important to you than the reason you're on the journey in the first place, you're likely to quit and head right back to your favorite spot on the couch.

This isn't to say that setting goals, such as a future race, is a bad idea. Quite the opposite, as this can help you focus your efforts. But you shouldn't rely solely on an endpoint to keep you going.

When your primary reason for running is to build your self-esteem with every step, that's really all the motivation you need to start moving. Consider each and every step a stitch in your scarf of self-confidence, and start knitting.

GETTING STARTED

Now that I've convinced you that running is a wonder drug, able to solve all your problems and give you the confidence you've always wanted, what next? Duh, it's time to run.

Cue the deluge of questions: Where should I run? When? How far? What happens when I get tired? Won't I get injured because I'm overweight? Should I sign up for a race? Where do I get cute running clothes that fit? Do I need a GPS watch? What the heck are compression tights? Why is running so *hard*?

Patience, grasshopper. All in good time.

Our first goal is to get you running consistently–because once you've got a few runs under your belt, you've built evidence that you are indeed a runner. And what do runners do? All together now ... *they run*! When you believe you're a runner, you are much more likely to get out there and do it. Which builds more evidence. It's the opposite of a vicious cycle–more like a self-confidence spiral, perhaps? Yes, that's what we'll call it. Imagine that each and every run you complete is a magical step in the spiral staircase to the glistening ivory tower of self-esteem.

Gag.

But seriously, consistency not only gets physical results like running faster and farther, it builds up your positive belief system. And the stronger those good feelings are, the more likely you are to keep running. So without further ado, let's begin.

Download this jumpstart plan and have it handy as you go through the next few sections so you can take notes and be ready to start off with confidence:

www.NotYourAverageRunner.com/start

DECISIONS, DECISIONS

The first question to tackle is where and when you should run. The short answer? Wherever and whenever you'll be most likely to actually do it. This means that if you love being outdoors in all four seasons, you might want to rethink putting that $5000 treadmill on layaway. But if you don't mind working out in your basement and have the latest season of your favorite show cued up on Netflix, a treadmill might be the right choice. Either way, I urge you to experiment a lot in the beginning to find what works for you. Run on your local roads or trails, at the gym, after you get up in the morning, and during your lunch break to see what you like best. There are pros and cons to every scenario, but the most important thing is that it is right for *you*.

CLIMATE CONTROLLED COMFORT OR THE GREAT OUTDOORS?

Ah, the great debate. Is it better to run on a treadmill, or brave the elements and head outside? A lot depends on your work and family schedules, where you live and, of course, personal preference. Most likely, no single option will be perfect – rather, you will find that a combination of places works best for you.

Let's consider the gym. Pros: convenience, quality of equipment, air-conditioning, and safety. In this day and age, many of us have a gym strategically located close to either work or home. Gyms usually have high-quality treadmills built for heavy use, which means they won't shake and shimmy when you push the speed past 3.5 mph. With a more cushioned surface than pavement or cement, the impact to your joints is lower. Another bonus of the treadmill is the incline, allowing you to run uphill when you want to. Most facilities even have TVs hanging from the ceiling (although in my experience, someone else is always in control of the remote, and they always want to watch golf). Gyms have locker rooms, which means you can shower right afterwards if you choose, as well as lock up your stuff while you're running. There is also the luxury of air-conditioning in the summer, heat in the winter, and a roof when it is raining. Unlike roads, treadmills are traffic-free, so you can crank up the tunes as loud as you want without fear of getting run over by someone texting and driving. Working out around other people that are also sweating, huffing and puffing can be motivational, and the hidden benefit here is that you can secretly race the person on the next machine (something I highly recommend).

Cons? Not too many, aside from cost and hygiene. Most gyms are not free. However, in recent years, low cost gyms have been popping up all over the place. If you're not looking for a space with lots of bells and whistles, you can probably get a membership someplace for less than $20 a month and no annual contract. So cost shouldn't be too much of a barrier. The questionable cleanliness of a public gym is the biggest drawback, in my opinion. Sure, *you* wipe down your equipment with disinfectant after use, and wash your hands after you leave the bathroom, *but not everyone does*. The residue of others' bodily fluids are on nearly every surface at a gym–the whole point of being there is to generate sweat– and you will eventually (and probably unknowingly) come into contact with someone else's bacterial and viral leftovers. Icky, yes. Also inevitable. So do your best not to put your hands in your mouth while you're there and make sure to shower pretty quickly after you're done. And if you're sick, stay home. Nobody else wants your germs.

If you prefer treadmill running, but don't want a full gym membership, consider getting a treadmill for your home. This is the ultimate in convenience, because unless the power goes out, you're guaranteed to be able to run. Actually, you can still get a workout even if there's no power–it takes a lot of strength to push the belt without electrical assistance, but it can be done (just ask my clients). Truth be told, it feels just like pushing a manual lawnmower up a steep hill, and that's a pretty awesome workout. A home treadmill session is also a great opportunity to catch up on your favorite movies or TV shows, and you don't have to fight anyone for the remote. Win-win!

Other than the boredom factor and up-front investment cost, there aren't too many cons about treadmills aside from one: running on a belt does not challenge your body the way running outdoors does, because the belt is doing some of the work for you by pulling your feet backwards. And if you're training for a race, this could be an issue. There is no wind resistance or terrain variability on a treadmill either, which is always a factor outside. To compensate, consider varying the incline and speed to better mimic outdoor conditions, if your goal is to complete a 5K or other event.

So that's the scoop on the indoors–now let's talk about what's outside the gym. Running outdoors has advantages and disadvantages too, but unlike your trusty treadmill, there are many more options. Unless you live in a tree house in the rainforest, outdoor running is convenient. Step out the front door and you're ready to roll. If your neighborhood is replete with sidewalks and well-manicured lawns, consider yourself lucky. You are in running heaven. Also, please consider inviting me over to be your running buddy. I'll bring my famous homemade granola bars.

Those of you that don't have miles of traffic-free streets and sidewalks just outside your front door need not fret, however, you'll just need to be a bit more careful: look both ways before crossing the street, be aware of approaching traffic, follow the rules of the road and watch for potholes or other obstacles. Whatever your road situation, pounding the pavement can be a tremendously joyous way to get your run on. Whether in the city, the country, or somewhere in between, running outside means you have a constantly changing landscape to watch, and although you will have to go uphill from time to time, that means you also get to enjoy the delights of going downhill. Since we live in such a traffic-centered society, roads are everywhere (sidewalks, not so much), thus there are infinite possibilities to wear out even the most tireless runner. And with all of the free online mapping tools available, you can plan out your route in detail ahead of time–or just throw caution to the wind and see where your feet take you.

The downsides to street and sidewalk running are few, but do need to be considered. The shoulders of most roads are sloped to allow for water runoff. This means that you'll constantly be running at a very slight angle which over time can result in muscle imbalances. To counteract this, make sure you don't do every run on this type of surface. Mix it up with sidewalks, trails and track running if possible. Traffic is also a big concern, and although rural roads tend to have fewer cars, this also means those vehicles that are on the road will be driving faster and probably not paying as close attention to the side of the road as might someone that is in heavier traffic. Always run facing oncoming traffic and stay aware. Be ready to duck and roll into a ditch if necessary. Wear appropriate reflective gear and brightly colored clothing at all times, but especially at dusk and after dark. Headlamps and blinking lights may look dorky, but if you want to run after sundown, they can be invaluable. It could mean the difference between a successful run or a ride to the hospital.

Pavement and cement can pose tripping hazards due to the potential for holes, cracks and uneven surfaces (especially if you live in Pennsylvania where the unofficial state flag is orange and says "Caution, Men Working"). Roads and sidewalks are also harder on the joints. Again, watch where you're going and make sure to mix up your surfaces and you should be fine.

The final challenge with running outdoors is the weather, and this is the one that most people complain about. Cold, heat, humidity and precipitation pose their own challenges, but unless there is lightning or hail (or the temp is below zero degrees Fahrenheit), there's no reason you can't suit up accordingly and soldier on.

By the way, running any given route in the rain makes you 50% more hardcore than running the very same route on a sunny day–which puts you several levels higher up the self-esteem spiral by default. Now that's something to consider!

Finally, let's talk track and trail. Tracks are awesome–no traffic, outside, and a nice cushy running surface. If you can find a nearby high school or college that will let you run on their track when the students aren't using it, you've got a fabulous training tool available to you. Bonus points if you can find one that is well-lit after dark! The only drawback to a track workout is the lack of hills (of course, to some this might be their best feature), and the fact that sometimes there are football games, track meets, or other activities going on that will take precedence over your need to run.

Trail running is incredible, but also much more demanding physically, due to the elastic nature of the ground. Ditto for running on grass. I won't go into the physics of it all, but the more "give" your running surface has, the harder your muscles have to work to keep you moving. This is a good thing overall because running on pavement will feel easy after you've trained on packed dirt or grass, but you'll definitely run slower in the woods. Watch for tree roots, gopher holes and small animals, and make sure you don't get poked in the eye by a stray branch. If at all possible, bring a map and tuck it into your pocket or a backpack. It's easy to ask for directions when you're lost in an unfamiliar neighborhood, but there usually aren't too many pedestrians in the woods at your local state park. GPS is your friend; use it if you have it. Finally, for a true trail run, you'll need sturdier running shoes, or at the very least a pair that you don't mind getting dirty. Check your local running store for recommendations.

THE BEST TIME TO RUN

Alrighty! Now that we've covered the where, what about the when? The best timing for your runs can be a bit trickier to nail down. It mainly depends on your schedule and whether you're a night owl or an early bird. If you're willing and able to get up an hour earlier, morning runs are a great way to make sure you fit it in as well as start your day off right. I'm not going to lie to you and say that running first thing is easy-peasy, but there are a few things you can do make the process less painful. Remove as many obstacles from your path as possible (or to look at it another way, create obstacles to staying in bed):

- Lay out your clothes the night before (or pack your gym bag and *put it in the car*).
- Put your alarm clock on the other side of the room so you actually have to get out of bed to turn it off.

- Go to bed a little early to make sure you're well-rested.
- Train your spouse to push you out of bed when the alarm goes off.
- If you have a running buddy, make a date so you know someone will be waiting for you–this works particularly well if said running buddy has no issues with publicly shaming you for not showing up.
- Make sure your phone and other devices are fully charged (or charging) before you go to bed.
- Keep your list of reasons why you run on your phone or in your nightstand, and review it if you want to sleep in.
- And my favorite trick of all, just get dressed. When the alarm goes off, tell yourself all you need to do is put on your workout clothes and shoes. Once that's done, tackle the next step.

If evening workouts are better for you, the same principles apply. Remove the barriers and excuses ahead of time:

- Pack your gym bag the night before and put it in the car.

- Keep a spare set of everything (clothes, sports bra, ponytail holder, sneakers, socks, even headphones) in your car.
- Run at work if possible, or choose a gym or trail that is on your way home.
- If you run in your neighborhood, get dressed to run at work–when you get home, don't even go in the house, just hop out of the car and start running.
- Listen to energizing music in the car on the way home from work to get yourself pumped up.
- Plan to meet a buddy for your run.

If you have a flexible work schedule, try running at lunch or another time during the day. And if you're an at-home mom with little ones, running strollers have come a long way–taking your child with you on your workout makes him happy too!

"I have an eleven-month-old son, so I have to take him with me most days. Getting my son outside and on the road motivates me to get out the door. He is a much happier little guy after a stroll. I have to work around nap times and make sure I take loops that keep me close to the house just in case he gets fussy. I think getting him moving and exposed to the fresh air is great for him, too."

–NINA G., CHERRY HILL, NJ

My client Janis even loads her three miniature dachshunds (she calls them 'the Weenies') into a running stroller so she can take them running with her.

The bottom line is, the only perfect time to run is the one that works for you. Consider your schedule, lifestyle, and personality and try out a few things. You'll need to experiment to find the best fit, but eventually you'll figure it out.

DEALING WITH THE WEATHER

Running on a treadmill has one distinct advantage over outdoor running: the climate indoors is usually a cool seventy degrees, with 0% chance of precipitation. If only the rest of the world was like that! But it isn't, and sooner or later you'll need to figure out how to deal with Mother Nature.

The height of summer is my least favorite time to run. I'm not a fan of the heat, so when the temperature and humidity get so high I wonder if I've been teleported to a rainforest, my first instinct is to turn up the air conditioning, lie on the couch and crack open a cold beer. With a little planning, however, running in the heat doesn't need to be a suffer-fest. Keep the following advice in mind and you'll be fine:

- Run early in the morning or late in the evening, when the temperatures are lower.
- Slow down. Heat and humidity are hard on your body. The more moisture in the air, the slower your sweat will evaporate. This means that you're much more prone to overheating–to avoid this, you'll need to ease up a bit on your pace and take some extra walk breaks. If you normally cover a mile in twelve minutes when the temperature is sixty degrees and dry, you might run a fourteen-minute mile on a humid, ninety degree day. This is normal, and doesn't mean you're losing fitness.
- Expose yourself. The more skin you have uncovered, the easier it will be to keep cool. This means sleeveless tops, and tights that don't go past your knees.
- Try a cooling towel or cooling shirt. These items get really cold when they get wet and can help you manage your body temperature on really hot days. My client Karen wore a cooling shirt to a race when it was nearly 100 degrees out, and the shirt worked

so well by the end she was actually chilly and had to put on a dry shirt to warm up!

- Wear a lightweight headband or a visor to keep sweat out of your eyes. Avoid hats, which trap heat.

- Don't apply sunscreen above your eyebrows. If you do this, you'll end up with sunscreen in your eyes, guaranteed.

- Drink water. Carrying a bottle with you while you run can be a hassle, so leave it next to a fencepost or tree that you'll pass by more than once on your route. If my stash-spot is in a high-traffic area, I usually tape a note to my bottle that says "Please don't take me. My owner is out running right now and is really looking forward to drinking me later!"

- Put ice cubes in your bra at the start of your run. I'm serious.

- If you find yourself overheating, dump water over your head. This is a really fast way to cool down.

- And finally, know the warning signs of heatstroke: chills, dizziness, muscle cramps, weakness and nausea. Always carry your phone in case you need to call for help.

Winter running is also a challenge, but still completely possible. Again, it's all about heat management. You might start out with your teeth chattering but after a few minutes of running your body temperature rises and suddenly that long-sleeved shirt and fleece jacket feel like a neoprene wetsuit. To avoid this scenario, dress yourself in light layers–especially on top–so that you can peel them off as your body warms up. One strategy I like to use is to leave my house with a jacket, run for five minutes or so until I'm warmed up, then swing back by my house and drop the jacket off in the mailbox. Don't forget about water, either. Dry, winter air causes your sweat to evaporate quickly, which means you'll need to replenish your fluids often.

No matter the season, you'll always have to deal with some sort of precipitation. There's really no reason not to run in the rain or snow (unless there's lightning, hail, or flash flooding in the area), but it can be uncomfortable if you're not prepared. You can wear a waterproof jacket, but just remember, if it keeps water off your body, it also traps any moisture you generate - which leads to chafing. So if you choose to run in the rain or snow (personally, I love it), plan on getting wet. Use extra BodyGlide on your feet and other body parts prone to chafing, and make sure to put your electronics in a water-proof case (or a plastic baggie). Keep an extra close eye on traffic, too–wet or icy roads can be slippery so stick to routes where you'll be far from moving vehicles.

EXPECT THE UNEXPECTED

Even the best-laid plans can fall apart sometimes, so it's important to have a backup strategy. If you're a die-hard trail runner, where will you run when the spring floods wash out your favorite path? What if you get to the gym and all the treadmills are taken? Will you run outdoors during your favorite seasons and indoors the rest of the year? What if, despite your best efforts, you sleep through your alarm? You'll need to determine how you will manage through those (inevitable) times when your preferred running option is unavailable. Otherwise, you might find yourself stomping around the house in frustration, wondering how many times you'd have to run up and down the stairs to cover one mile.

For the record, one mile of stairs equals 528 trips up and 528 trips back down, based on a standard staircase with 15 steps. I don't even know how long that would take, and I'd rather run an entire marathon on a treadmill than find out.

My point is, if you fail to plan, you plan to fail. Think ahead, remove as many obstacles as possible, and you'll rarely miss a workout due to unforeseen circumstances. The more workouts you finish, the higher you climb on your self-esteem spiral.

YOUR INNER MEAN GIRL

When you first start running, you will experience all manner of new sensations in your body. In particular, your legs, feet, knees, hips, back, lungs … almost everywhere. Including your brain! Training your mind to run is just as tough (perhaps even more so) than your body, regardless of your weight or fitness level.

Many of these new feelings will be uncomfortable, perhaps even painful. As I've said before, running is hard work, and it takes time to adapt. So you might be tempted to interpret these phenomena as a warning sign from your body that it is time to take a rest break. With a Snickers bar.

In a nutshell, your body is a lot like the government. When the going gets tough, there is often a lot of hand-waving, pounding of fists, and threats of a shutdown. But with a little coaxing and negotiating, eventually everyone settles down and things continue operating as normal.

The trick is to learn the difference between actual pain, which should be respected and tended, and your inner mean girl, who is just trying to convince you that you suck. Yeah, she's a bully. She's also relentless, unless you learn how to handle her.

When I'm running and a thought like "I want to stop" pops into my head, I use a body-scanning technique to figure out what to do. Fortunately, the body scan can be done while running, and doesn't require any special equipment. Starting with my toes and slowly working my way upwards ... feet, heels, calves, shins, knees, thighs, hips, spine, chest, back, shoulders, neck ... to the very top of my head, I look for actual pain, such as a sharp, stabbing feeling, anything that feels like pulling, popping or tearing (tearing is always bad), or a deep ache that appears to be getting worse. These are usually signs that something is amiss, and running through these signals can lead to injury. When you feel the urge to stop due to potential pain, you'll need to hone right in on the sensations to see if the pain is real or imaginary. Often when you focus all your attention on the body part in question, the feeling disappears. This is how you know your mean girl is up to her old shenanigans.

Of course, if you detect true pain, please stop (or at least slow down), assess, and take appropriate action. If what you're feeling is general fatigue, weariness, boredom, or disappears when you focus on it, you might be a victim of mean girl mischief. This is great news for you, because I'm going to teach you how to kick her to the curb so you can keep going.

It will help enormously if you can give your mean girl a name. Trust me, this will make conversations with her much easier. And you will need to talk to her, or rather *stand up to her*. She's just a playground bully and when you hold your ground, she'll back down, I promise.

As I mentioned earlier, I call my mean girl Whinona. This is because she whines a *lot*, and her voice in my head is high pitched, nasal, and piercing. Also, because I don't personally know anyone called Winona, I felt comfortable that I wouldn't insult any of my friends or family by appropriating that name. But if your mean girl reminds you of your ninth grade frenemy, or your mother-in-law, feel free to use that name! It will be our little secret.

Sometimes Whinona starts in on me before I've even put my shoes on:

"You worked really hard yesterday. You need to rest."

"Let's just wait to see what kind of wine Hoda & Kathie Lee are drinking on the Today Show. Then we'll go."

"All of your workout clothes are in the laundry."

And my personal favorite:

"Nap first. Run later."

This one is always a lie. What she really means is "Nap first, cookie later, then we'll watch some Netflix."

The best defense is a good offense, and after years of practice, I'm now fully prepared with an arsenal of short and sweet rebuttals. Here's an example of a recent conversation:

This is hard. (You're right. Keep moving.)

I don't want to. (Your opinion is noted. Keep moving.)

You're running too slow. (So what? Keep moving.)

My legs are tired. (Awesome! That means we're working hard! Keep moving.)

That woman is staring at you (Must be because I'm so awesome. Keep moving.)

This hurts. (So does being out of shape. Keep moving.)

My toe hurts. (Let me check...sorry, it's not that bad. Keep moving.)

I'm bored. (Really? This is a great time to meditate, write a blog post in your head, see if you can remember all fifty states, work on your breathing, plan a vacation, look at the landscaping in your neighborhood for ideas …)

You look ridiculous. You're sweaty, red-faced, and panting like a porn star. (Well duh, that's what people look like when they run.)

You're too fat to run. (Really? Because I *am* running.)

I'm tired. (Me too–tired of hearing you whine. Shut up so I can finish this run.)

You get the picture. Arguing with her always makes things worse–the key is to listen to her complaints and acknowledge them, then respond calmly, logically, without getting emotional, and definitely without allowing further discussion on the topic.

A word of warning: she will almost certainly try to convince you that it is much harder to run if you're overweight, and that you might injure yourself. While she has a fair point, in my opinion she is playing to your emotions. An overweight woman has more body mass to move than someone that weighs less, that much is true. She also has correspondingly stronger legs from moving that very same weight around day in and day out, which somewhat compensates for the extra load. Regardless, it will take more effort and probably a longer training program for a woman that weighs 250 pounds to be able to run a 5K or half marathon than one who is starting at 150 pounds. But that's where it ends. All new runners, regardless of size or fitness level have the same mental hurdles to overcome and the same mean girl to vanquish, which really equalizes the playing field. If you work at your current ability, heed the warning signs of injury, and keep a consistent schedule, you'll get stronger. It doesn't matter if it takes you two months or two years, because if you stay focused on the reasons you run (which hopefully include building up your self-esteem), it won't matter how long it takes, all it will matter is that you keep doing it.

Working through the physical and mental discomfort of running can actually be rewarding, despite what your version of Whinona might tell you. Pain is inevitable, but suffering is optional. Listening to your mean girl is suffering. Don't give her the satisfaction.

NOW WHAT?

Now that you've figured out where and when to run, and how to shut down your inner mean girl like a boss, you're probably wondering how far and fast you should run. That is, of course, a great question, but since there are hundreds of books, websites and apps out there to tell you how to do just that, I'm not going to explore that topic in too much detail here. The purpose of this book is to show you that you can become a runner in the body you have right now—and to help you build self-esteem along the way.

That being said, I do have a few words to say on the topic. The kindest thing you can do for yourself is to start off slowly, by doing walk-run intervals at a pace that feels difficult, but not impossible. Depending on your current fitness level, this might mean you start with a thirty-minute workout, where you run for fifteen seconds and walk for sixty, or it might mean you run for two minutes and walk for thirty seconds to recover. It doesn't matter where you start, just that you keep at it and test your boundaries a bit during each workout. Running is hard work. If it feels easy, you're probably not pushing hard enough. Conversely, if you spend your entire workout feeling like you're about to see your breakfast again, you might be going too hard. Aim to spend a decent chunk of your running time in the sweet spot between effort and ease. It takes practice, but with time you'll get there. Using the body scan technique I described earlier will help you with that.

Whichever training plan you choose, just remember that everyone's body is different, and while these plans are created for the average person, they don't necessarily take *your* individual needs into account. If you are having trouble progressing to the next week in your training schedule, this doesn't mean you are a failure! It just means you need to adapt the plan to meet your needs.

The most important thing is to stick with it, go at your own pace, and be insanely proud of everything you complete.

To get you started, I've created a free beginner's guide, which you can find here:

www.NotYourAverageRunner.com/start

THE NEXT PHASE

You've accomplished quite a bit so far: settling into a comfortable routine and creating backup plans for your backup plans. All that's left to do is run your butt off and watch yourself get faster and faster each week, right?

Oops. About that … I've got some bad news.

There's no doubt that a running program is new and exciting at the start, when each week brings measurable improvement, and you can barely wait for the next workout to find out what your body can do. The awesome thing about this phase is that rapid gains in speed, distance or duration keep you thirsty for more, and build up your self-esteem tremendously. Each workout is an opportunity to push yourself just a little farther, and you'll often find that you exceed your own expectations. This is the honeymoon phase of running and it feels spectacular. Visions of entering a marathon dance in your head, and you realize that you are, in fact, a bona fide superhero. With a cape, and possibly even an invisible plane.

Beginners tend to see results faster than experienced runners, because they're starting, well, right at the beginning. During your first week as a runner, you might run fifteen second intervals interspersed with 2 minutes of walking, but after a few workouts, you'll realize you can double that time to a 30 seconds–a 100% increase in performance. A month or so later and you're running a minute at a time, doubling your endurance yet again. Fast forward three months, and you're consistently doing 3 miles of intervals with ease, running at least half the time. Amazing! Your days of running fifteen seconds are a distant memory, but the delight of doubling your running time in a matter of days is still fresh in your mind.

Now that you're conquering longer runs with ease, adding an interval or two to the length of your runs seems insignificant. For example, ramping up from twenty to twenty-two intervals is a 10% improvement, which is a great return on investment if you're saving for retirement, but doesn't seem quite so glamorous to a new runner, who is used to 100% gains every few weeks. You should know, however, that 10% is a *huge* improvement in the world of elite runners, and can mean the difference between taking home the gold or not getting a medal. It's all about perspective.

Regardless, once the honeymoon is over, you'll need to look at the big picture, rather than a weekly snapshot, to see a noticeable change. We've talked at length about finding the underlying reasons you run, and keeping them in mind on those days when you want to roll over and go back to sleep. But it also helps to cultivate a few extra reasons–such as short or long-term goals, or an accountability partner, to get you through the tough times.

There are any number of ways to keep yourself interested and your routine feeling fresh and new—the only limit is your imagination. Consider your personality, fitness goals, and lifestyle: Are you someone that likes delayed gratification, or do you prefer immediate rewards? Do you like to count down the days to an event, or let your rewards build up over time? Do you crave group interaction, or are you a lone wolf?

Instant gratification junkies are motivated by a quick hit of success. The trick is to choose something that is easily achievable in the near future so it holds your interest. For example, if you're able to do a half-mile now, strive to finish a mile (then two, then three, etc). If you can cover a mile in 14 minutes, work towards running it in 13 minutes. You get the picture.

Other ideas:

- Begin adding 0.5 mph to your regular treadmill speed for one interval, then build up to running all your intervals at the new speed.
- Make it up that really tough hill on your regular route without stopping to rest.

- Pick a nearby destination and work up to running there from your house.
- Find someone running ahead of you and catch up to them.
- On a track, see how fast you can complete one lap, then try to beat your time.

If you savor the process of achieving a goal more than the goal itself, choose something that is farther in the future, such as a race. Or get creative:

- Work towards accumulating distance over time, such as 100 miles in a month.
- Get a wall map of your state, plot a course to run from edge to edge, and track your progress on the map. (If you live in Rhode Island, this might be more of a short-term goal.)
- Put $1 in a jar after every run and work towards a specific savings target. Reward yourself with something fun like a massage or a cute running outfit when you hit it. Or treat me with something fun! It's always better to give than receive, right?
- Pick a race and train for it (more about that later).

- Keep a journal describing each run, however you see fit. Include your distance, time, weather, how you felt, what you thought about, things you saw along the route–whatever is meaningful to you.
- Set up a series of mini-goals that take you incrementally towards a bigger achievement.
- Chart your progress using a spreadsheet or a big wall chart. This helps you visualize just how much you've accomplished (and it's just plain fun, for Post-it Note nerds like me).

Of course, not everybody is concerned with going faster or farther. If you couldn't care less about your running stats and just want to spice things up a bit, here are some ideas that are focused more on fun than progress:

- Try a new route each week.
- Mix up your running playlist.
- Wear a tutu to your next race (I'm only partly joking– this is an actual thing. Google it.)
- Break up the monotony by incorporating strength training into your runs: stop for body-weight or resistance band exercises in between running intervals.

- Literally run errands. Run to the library, post office, drug store. Save gas and get your workout in! Just don't buy eggs. It's no fun to run home with eggs in your backpack.
- High-five everyone you pass.
- Run backwards for short distances (but only if you're in a safe area, like a track).
- Incorporate thirty-second intervals of skipping–fun, silly and challenging.

Another sure-fire way to keep the mojo alive is to get pumped up with music. Getting lost in the beat can make the minutes and miles fly by. The best songs inspire me to pick up my pace, keep going a little longer, or power up a tough hill when I'd rather walk. Dance, hip hop and techno tunes seem to work best for me, but whatever music gets your toes tapping will do the job. One trick I use is to reserve my favorite songs for my runs, and refrain from listening to them at other times–this makes me excited to put on my sneakers, because I know the dance party in my head is about to start. If you're a treadmill runner, try this same strategy with your favorite TV shows or movies. Avid reader? Load up your phone with an audiobook.

Just don't read on the treadmill. It's almost impossible to run and read, and you might find yourself tripping and flying off the back of the machine if you try. Entertainment for everyone else, but pretty painful for you. So save the books and magazines for the recumbent bike, unless you want to end up in a YouTube video of fitness fails.

YOU'VE GOT A FRIEND

Running can be a great opportunity to spend time with friends or meet new people, and can help you stay motivated. Whether you're on a trail or side-by-side treadmills at the gym, running with a buddy has a million advantages (well, maybe not a million, but definitely a lot):

- Bonding: Catch up on each other's lives (and all the juicy gossip) without the extra calories of a margarita or a triple-foam latte.
- Accountability: Knowing someone is counting on you to be there for a workout (and that they'll be pretty annoyed if you don't show up) is a pretty strong motivator.
- Encouragement: Having someone to commiserate with when the going gets tough can mean the

difference between quitting halfway through or finishing strong.

And it's just plain fun to run with someone else!

For outdoor runs, try to choose a partner that runs at a similar ability, and lay out the ground rules ahead of time–choose a pace, distance and interval schedule that allows each of you to get the workout you need. It might be a slow day for one of you and a fast day for the other, or perhaps you'll do the first half of the run together and finish separately.

A few words of warning about the buddy plan: running (and exercise in general) can decrease your inhibitions, and sometimes there is a tendency to, how shall I say this, *overshare* after you're all warmed up and have run out of gossip. Sure, finding out that your bestie leads a double-life as an exotic dancer will keep you running for a few extra miles, but she needs to know that her secret is safe with you. Don't break the code. Whatever happens on the run, stays on the run.

If you prefer a group environment, check out your local running stores–they often have free groups that run after work or on weekend mornings. Before you show up for your first run, however, be sure to ask the right questions of the organizer. The website might say that all levels are welcome, but if their idea of a beginning runner is a twelve-minute-per-mile pace and you're running much slower than that, you're going to set yourself up to feel pretty bad when the group takes off and you end up running by yourself for most of the workout. Find out who leads the runs, what the general pace is, if there's anyone designated to stay behind and keep track of stragglers. It also helps to understand what the route will be like. Will you be running on sidewalks, trails, or high traffic areas? Is the terrain flat or hilly? How many miles are covered in a typical outing? Are there options to do a shorter loop? What happens if you get lost?

If you can't find a group that meets your needs at your local running store, check out Meetup.com or a similar site to find people at your ability, or consider a virtual running club.

Psst - the best virtual running group on the internet is the Not Your Average Runner group on Facebook, with thousands of women exactly like you.

Join here:
www.NotYourAverageRunner.com/jointhecommunity

What if you're someone that needs a little individual attention, or you can't find a running group that meets your needs? Consider a running coach, someone who knows how to keep you motivated and accountable, and will create a training program that is customized to your individual needs. Coaches aren't just for experienced athletes, either. Most beginners can benefit from getting proper instruction from the very beginning, to avoid injury, stay motivated, learn how to run the right way, and most importantly have fun doing it!

Just because the honeymoon is over doesn't mean the fun has to stop. Finding ways to keep the love alive ensures that you'll have a long, happy relationship with your new sport.

And if, despite all of the above, you find yourself taking a few months (or even years) off from running, don't despair! It took me 15 years to make my running habit stick. You can always start up again. That's the beautiful thing about running–it will always be there for you, waiting patiently for your return.

"I read a "Marathons for Dummies" book several years ago. It claimed that there was no such thing as "jogging." If you are not walking then you are running. That stuck with me. I am not a fast runner, but I am a runner. I often tell people, "I may not have speed but I have endurance." There are periods when I run every day, periods when I run a couple of times a week, and even sometimes when I don't run at all, but I am still a runner."

-McKenzie D., Bend, Oregon

RUNNERS GONNA RUN

Everyone has that person in their life that feels the need to rain on your parade. Actually, you're pretty fortunate if it's *only* one person. They're basically your inner mean girl come to life - dropping comments designed to make you feel worse and themselves feel superior. These people are rarely runners–we're a pretty positive and supportive bunch, and we love new recruits–but they might have tried to become a runner in the past and failed. Regardless, your success and joy with your new sport makes them feel worse about themselves, so they'll try to discourage you from pursuing your dream:

"You're going to destroy your knees."

"Real runners don't take walk breaks."

"You're just a jogger, not a runner."

"Running is dangerous–I heard about a guy who had a heart attack while doing a marathon last year!"

"Don't you get bored? Running is just so boring!"

Yeah, yeah, yeah. Everyone has an opinion, and they're entitled to speak it. But the only way someone else's opinions can hurt you is if you believe them–so don't! Recognize their words for what they are–a reflection on the speaker, not you. The easiest way to deal with this type of person is to simply say "thanks for your concern," and change the subject. Haters gonna hate. It's human nature. Fortunately, runners gonna run.

Once you've learned how to deal with the external haters, you might find that your mean girl has a few more tricks up her sleeve. Whinona loves to compare me to others, and in the absence of that, to myself.

Looking at how fast, far, or frequently someone else runs, how much weight she's lost from running, how much cuter her outfit is than yours–basically anything that leaves you feeling "*less than*" in any way, is poisonous. Nothing can kill your self-esteem faster than comparing yourself to someone else's success and deciding that you are a failure. I don't mean using someone else as an example of what is possible– that's actually an awesome way to improve yourself. No, I mean using someone else's success to beat yourself up for not being good enough. The worst part is, you might not even realize you're doing it. Whenever I hear someone say "That was a terrible run. I should have run much faster" or "I can't keep up with everyone else, so I'm not even going to try," my heart breaks a little. I also get kinda pissed off at their mean girl.

Other people's performance is their business. It is a result of their hard work, yes, but also a result of how they felt that day, the weather, their internal self-talk, what they ate for breakfast, how much sleep they got, and a million other factors. It has nothing to do with you and in no way reduces your accomplishment.

The same goes for how you ran last week, last month, or last year vs. today. Some days the stars align and the experience is nothing short of euphoric, while other days it will be a battle just to get out the door. This is completely normal! As I mentioned above, if you track your performance over months–not days or weeks–you'll see improvement. Realize that developing a running habit takes time (heck, it took me almost fifteen years to make mine stick!) and that you might even go months at a time without running. This is also completely normal, and, I would venture to say, probably a good thing, because it allows you to appreciate the differences in your body and mind when you're running regularly and when you're not. Eventually, the discomfort of not running will be greater than the discomfort of running. That's when you'll know you've got a lifetime habit.

Find the good in every single run, even if it is as simple as saying "I ran today."

TAKING IT TO THE NEXT LEVEL

"In running, it doesn't matter whether you come in first, in the middle of the pack, or last. You can say, 'I have finished.' There is a lot of satisfaction in that."

–FRED LEBOW, CO-FOUNDER, NEW YORK CITY MARATHON

D id you know that women weren't allowed to participate in the track and field portion of the Olympics until 1928? And that the first women's Olympic marathon wasn't held until 1988? As ridiculous as it sounds today, at the time running was considered too strenuous for women. Fortunately for you and I, things have changed a lot since then–women now represent a sizable portion of the field in any footrace, and we are kicking butt.

Should you give racing a try? In my opinion, yes. To start with, a race can be a lot of fun. It's the ultimate group workout, with people lining the streets to cheer you on, plus you always get a free t-shirt! As a motivational tool, knowing that you have to run a specific distance on a specific date can't be beat. And when those annoying runners in your office can't stop talking about their weekend activities, you'll finally have something to contribute to the conversation.

But really, a race is the perfect opportunity to push your limits and really see what you're capable of achieving. The thrill of running with a crowd of like-minded humans, all going in the same direction, striving together to achieve the same goal is simply incredible. A primal instinct you didn't even know you had is activated, and the energy of the group elevates you to new levels. If you didn't feel like a runner before your first race, you'll definitely feel like one afterwards.

What can you expect your first time? A lot depends on the distance and the number of people running. Shorter races, such as 1-mile "fun runs" or 5K (five kilometers, or 3.1 miles) distances tend to attract smaller crowds and have fewer runners. A local 5K might have as few as twenty-five entrants, but if it is a popular event, that number might be 1,000 or more. In a shorter race, you're also likely to encounter a combination of runners and walkers, especially for charity events, and the atmosphere is usually very relaxed and supportive.

Mid-to-long-distances, such as the half-marathon (13.1 miles) or marathon (26.2 miles) tend to be larger events, especially in major metropolitan areas. Expect the number of runners to be well over 1,000, and commonly over 10,000. Well-established events such as the New York Marathon are so popular that a lottery system has been established to ensure everyone has a fair chance to snag one of the 47,000 spots at the starting line. And no, that's not a typo. Forty-seven thousand people, all running simultaneously, for 26.2 miles. Thousands upon thousands of spectators turn out to watch, making the experience truly memorable for everyone. It's definitely on my bucket list.

If you love the idea of a timed race, but don't relish the thought of running with hundreds or thousands of other people by your side (or you live in a part of the country where races are hard to find) consider a virtual race - an event that allows you to run your distance where and when you want, and still get an awesome finisher's medal!

Perhaps you don't care for the idea of being timed, but still want the joy of running with others? Consider joining the recent trend of 5K run/walk events where there is no clock, such as a color run. These activities are pretty much just a big party disguised as a workout: fun and sweaty, with snacks. You still get the t-shirt along with a lot of great memories, but nobody keeps track of how long it took you to cross the finish line.

Before you sign up for your first event, do your research on seasonal weather, terrain, distance, location, size and rules. Almost every race has its own website with this information. Ask around (or do an online search) for anyone else that has run it in the past, to find out if it has typically been well-organized.

Choose a training plan based on your current fitness level, then stick to it as much as possible (if you need help finding a good plan, I've included a free chapter from my book *Not Your Average 5K* at the end of this book!). Think of training for a race like studying for a test. Cramming it all in the night before won't result in your best performance, and the same goes for a 5K. Do your homework, study a little every week, and you'll be much happier with the final outcome. I like to think of a race as a really fun reward for all the hard work I've done in the previous weeks and months. But don't worry too much about whether you've picked the perfect training schedule. The human body responds to physical stress by getting stronger, and for beginners, almost any consistent and progressive plan will work.

The most challenging part of your training will be mental. Sometimes, after weeks, or even months, of training, it can start to feel a lot like a job. A really sweaty job with no pay and no dental plan. When this happens, allow yourself to rediscover the joy of running by giving yourself permission to take a break. Missing a couple workouts (not ten) does not mean you'll lose strength and endurance–quite the opposite, in fact. Taking a short rest during a long training plan can often translate into better performance, better sleep, and higher quality workouts in the end.

Throughout your training, it is also likely that you'll feel nervous, worried, and anxious about race day. This is completely normal, even for veteran runners. Ask yourself why you are nervous. If you're worried about finishing, you have no need to be concerned. You will definitely finish. You've been training for weeks, possibly months, and you know you can go the distance. If it gets too hard, you'll slow down. You've got this.

Are you worried about finishing in a certain time? Stop right there. If this is your first race, whatever time you get will be a personal record. If not, try to understand why that particular time is so important to you, and what you think that means if you fail. Does it take away from the achievement of running this race? No. Does it take away from the achievement of training for this race? No. Does it mean you aren't a fit, healthy, amazing woman? Again, no. It just means that on that day, in those circumstances, that's how fast you ran. Nothing more, nothing less. You can always try again.

If you are concerned about what other people will think about your time, you are wasting your thoughts and creating unnecessary pain for yourself. Other people will think what they want and you can't do anything about it–the only thing you can control is your own mind. And really, most of them are probably thinking "Wow, I wish I could do that." So relax, slow down, and enjoy the process. The race is just the icing on the cake. The real work is what you're doing right now. And you're working your butt off, so be proud!

When race day comes, make sure you've double-checked the race rules. There are usually requirements for placement of your number, whether you can wear headphones, and where to place your timing chip, to name a few. If you don't follow them, you risk being disqualified.

Get to the starting line at least a half-hour early to hit up the Port-a-Potties and assess the situation. If you're slow, you'll want to start at the back of the pack. Nothing feels worse than hearing the starting gun go off and feeling the pressure of hundreds of people trying to push past you all at once. Larger races will corral you by anticipated race pace, and start you off in waves to make sure that everyone gets a fair chance. Don't worry about being too far back–you can always pass people later as the field thins out! And it feels a lot better to catch up to other people than it does to have everyone in the entire race pass you by. Fact.

Once you've crossed the starting line, the race is yours to enjoy. Savor each moment, connect with the fans, talk to others along the route, and encourage everyone you see, especially if they seem to be struggling. And if it happens to be you in last place, who cares? Finishing is finishing, regardless of how long it took. There is no shame in the back of the pack. Just remember to smile for the camera as you cross the finish line!

And speaking of the back of the pack, I have a personal story to share about one of my favorite races: the 2003 Presidential Run in Reading, Pennsylvania, a small 5K with only about fifty people. At the time, I had been running consistently for over a year, and was looking forward to seeing what I could do. My husband decided to join me for moral support and as we lined up at the start, I surveyed the rest of the runners, most of whom looked pretty experienced. There were no other chunky monkeys like me, but I did notice a much older woman dressed in a purple track suit and thought "Yes. I am going to Take. Her. Down."

The gun went off, and within about two minutes, I was dead last. The woman in purple left me in the dust! It was a tiny bit humiliating (especially after I found out she was almost forty years older than me) but overall I was pretty happy just to be running on that autumn day. The weather was beautiful–cold, crisp and clear–and the course was on a lovely trail next to the Schuylkill River. As I approached the finish line, at approximately forty-two minutes, my husband kindly slowed down so that I wouldn't be in last place. That's the real spirit of running. And the woman in purple? I still think of her to this day, as an example of what is possible. In forty years, that will be me (but my track suit will be hot pink).

DRESS FOR SUCCESS

If you dress like a runner, you'll feel like a runner. I'm not saying you need to buy $200 running shoes, or those ridiculous shorts that are slit so far up the side you can see tan lines. I just mean that if you wear clothes designed for running, you'll be a lot more comfortable, which will help you stay motivated to keep doing it. Also, have you ever heard the phrase "fake it til you make it"? That applies here. Dress the part long enough, and you'll start to believe it.

Beginners tend to wear whatever is already in the closet. This might be a big baggy T-shirt and sweats, or it might be a foxy little spandex number with matching leg warmers leftover from your Jazzercise days …

No? Just me? OK, then, moving on.

It is completely normal to hesitate before investing in a new wardrobe for a habit you're not even sure you want to maintain, but after a few runs, it's time to take the plunge. You might even realize that running is a fantastic excuse to go shopping. The problem is, it's really easy to spend a fortune on gear that seemed like a good idea at the time, but ends up at the back of your closet after a couple workouts. Hopefully, this chapter will help you avoid some of those rookie mistakes, and all of your purchases will become well-used favorites over time.

Before we get too far into this discussion, however, I need to warn you–there will be some tough love ahead, as well as some frank discussion about the challenges of dressing a larger body for running. Some of you might feel anxiety, or perhaps even righteous anger while reading the next few pages. Please take my words in the spirit they are intended, which is to help you pump up your self-esteem and body confidence, feel great while you run, and simplify your life.

The first lesson? Stop using your clothes to hide your body when you run, and quit worrying about what others think. Nobody else is looking at you while you run. Seriously. Most people are far too concerned about themselves to give you even a passing glance–they are thinking about their own workout, when that cute guy is going to call, or where to go for dinner. Unless you're wearing a sequined bodysuit and matching tutu or singing along to Beyoncé at the top of your lungs, nobody cares.

LOCK AND LOAD

When you run, your breasts move up and down as well as side to side. For you lucky A and B cups out there, this is mostly just an inconvenience. But if you're a C or higher, all of that extra motion can cause back pain and throw your gait out of whack. That's why a sports bra is arguably the most important piece of running gear any woman needs. If you don't take any other advice I've given you in this book, heed this: your girls need proper support when you run. And by that I mean: Strap. Them. Down. Otherwise, they're going to fly around like a Baywatch lifeguard running down the beach in a bikini. Bouncing boobs might look sexy on TV, but in real life, they hurt. Big or small, if they're not properly immobilized when you're moving, you're going to suffer.

Unfortunately, good support isn't cheap. Expect to pay upwards of $50 if you have a lot on top. And here's more bad news: an effective sports bra is often about fit and function, with fashion trailing a distant third. Oh, the sacrifices we make for this sport! But unless you're planning to run shirtless, nobody will know what your bra looks like.

Invest in a few really good bras and take good care of them, and they will last you a long time. Choose one made primarily from a synthetic blend (with little to no cotton) that doesn't have much too much stretch (stretch equals bounce), and make sure it is rated as a motion-control bra. Padded, wide straps are best for larger breasts, while smaller girls can get away with racerback, pullover styles. Get measured (or follow the instructions on the website) to make sure you're getting the right size. If you're spilling out of it everywhere, this defeats the purpose. More coverage means more control. Personally, I won't run in anything but an Enell–if it's good enough for Oprah, it's good enough for me! While it won't win any style awards–think "straight jacket meets corset" –when I'm wearing one of these treasures, it feels as if a weight has literally been lifted off my chest. It's that effective. Moving Comfort has a great line too, and if you do an online search for "motion control bra" you'll find plenty of options.

And just in case you're not fully convinced, here's a cautionary tale: A few years back, I joined a friend in a 5K Mother's Day run. The morning of the race, she said that she planned to walk most of it, so I opted not to wear my trusty Enell, and instead wore a regular bra. However, when the adrenaline of the event kicked in, so did her running mojo – and she took off like a shot. She's 5'10" with loooong legs, so I was hustling like a madwoman just to keep up. I'm sure you can imagine the frenetic (and painful) bouncing that ensued. We crossed the finish line at a full-out sprint, and the camera captured me smiling from ear to ear, in mid bounce, left breast up high, right one down low. It is one of the funniest photos I've ever seen of myself, and a solid reminder that a good sports-bra is critical.

IF THE SHOE FITS

Shoes are the next most important decision. Choosing the perfect running shoe is not easy. Everyone's foot is different, and adding even more complexity to the issue is the question of what kind of runner you are. Do you over- or under-pronate? Are you a heel-striker or do you land more towards the ball of your foot? How much do you weigh? Do you prefer a soft cushy shoe or one with a more minimalist feel? There too many factors at play to allow me to offer succinct advice on how to choose the perfect shoe for you, so instead I'm going to refer you to your local running store. They're the experts.

A reputable brick-and-mortar store will measure your feet, analyze your gait, and discuss your weekly mileage and typical running surfaces before making a recommendation. In addition, they should allow you to run a short distance in the shoes, perhaps around the parking lot or on a treadmill in the store. And most importantly, they will accept returns. Running shoes are not cheap! You need to know that you have the option to bring them back and exchange for something else if it just doesn't work out. Ask a lot of questions, and understand the store policies before you buy. Online merchants, such as RoadRunner.com, have incredibly generous return policies, great prices and a huge selection.

A word of caution about the minimalist shoe trend that is currently sweeping the running world: although they are a great concept, this type of shoe is not always the friend of a heavier girl. If you've spent most of your exercise time in traditional sneakers, your ankles and feet might not be strong enough to handle the lack of support in this type of running shoe–and you might find yourself quickly sidelined with a painful overuse injury such as plantar fasciitis. Believe me, you do *not* want to deal with that! If you're interested, do your research into this type of shoe first, and if you decide to go forward with a pair, introduce them very slowly to your routine. Make sure to include lots of ankle and foot strengthening exercises (done in your bare feet) on your strength training days, and wear supportive shoes at all other times. You'll thank me later.

And while we're on the topic of footwear, let's talk about socks. Most of the time, socks are an afterthought, but they're actually pretty important! If they are too big or too small, too thick or too thin, you can end up with blisters. If they're 100% cotton, and you tend to have sweaty feet, you'll end up with ... you guessed it, blisters again. Blisters hurt, and when your feet hurt, you stop running.

Good socks are worth the extra cash, and in the grand scheme of things they're not a huge investment. Your local running store can guide you to the ones that will work for you. Plan to spend around $10-15 a pair and pick up at least three so you can get a week's worth of runs before you need to wash them.

YOU'RE NOT FOOLING ANYONE

When it comes to workout clothes, and running gear in particular, wearing stuff that fits properly is critical. Why? Because if it isn't comfortable, your workout will suck. You'll either be messing around with your clothes the whole time, trying to adjust them to feel right, or you'll be so miserable that you'll quit early. Also, nobody wants to see you picking a wedgie on the treadmill. Seriously. Don't be that person.

Make sure your clothes fit your *current* body–not the body you wish you had, or one that is three sizes larger than you are right now. It really doesn't matter how fabulous that neon racerback tank is, if your ta-tas are threatening to fly out of it with every step, your run is going to be a short one. Save that stuff for Zumba.

Most of the fit issues I've seen are of the "If I wear a ginormous shirt and baggy sweats, nobody will know I'm fat" variety. While I appreciate not wanting to wear clothes that cling like plastic wrap to your least favorite body parts, going too big is definitely *not* the answer. Too much fabric, especially 100% cotton, gets in the way of proper movement, bunches up in unpleasant places, and traps heat and moisture. Poorly fitted garments can also mean a lot of skin-to-skin contact–such as between thighs, or between your upper arms and the side of your body. All that rubbing ultimately leads to chafing, which causes painful, red welts on your skin. Chafing sucks. If your sweat can't evaporate properly, your skin will get rubbed raw, and this may keep you from running. Later on, I'll go into more detail on how to prevent chafing, but it starts with wearing clothes that fit.

Here's more tough love: if you think those huge t-shirts that hang to your knees make you look smaller, you're mistaken. You're not fooling anyone aside from yourself. Instead of camouflaging your size, they emphasize the biggest parts of your body. Dressing this way also shouts to the world that you're ashamed of your body. Is that really the message you want to send? Drop the security blanket and rock your curves. Wear a short-sleeved shirt, or (gasp!) a tank top, and let your knees see the light of day! You are beautiful and amazing exactly the way you are right now. Show others that you care about yourself by choosing clothes that fit.

And speaking of your knees, we need to talk about tights. What you wear on your bottom half is possibly even more important than the top. Simply put, if you wear yoga pants, loose shorts, or sweatpants to run, you leave yourself open to chafing from the seams between your thighs. Anything that doesn't hug your legs is going to ride up, which means you'll spend a lot of time tugging them back down. It sucks, and it's completely avoidable if you wear running tights. They fit like a glove and move with you instead of rubbing against your skin, which will save you a lot of pain and suffering. I know you're cringing right now at the thought of wearing something so form-fitting in public, but you're going to have to trust me on this one. Tights come in several different lengths, from mid-thigh to ankle, so you should have no problem finding something that suits you. And here's some great news: they actually make you look thinner, because they don't add bulk. They also keep jiggling to a minimum while you're moving. Pair your tights with a shirt that hits below your hips if you're concerned about covering your tummy or butt. And if you're still feeling over-exposed, consider a running skirt, which combines tights with a skirt that hangs to mid-thigh. These have been rising in popularity lately with several manufacturers offering really cute options.

SHOP TIL YOU DROP

Before you hop in your car to head to the mall, you'll need to think about where you're most likely to find your size range. If you're a size L or smaller, you'll be able to shop anywhere, but those of you that wear an XL or larger may have to look a little harder. Personally, I find this to be somewhat ironic. Society tells us that we need a thin body to be accepted, but then makes it difficult to find cute clothing appropriate to do the very activity that will help us get there. It's maddening.

Fortunately, over the past few years, several forward-thinking companies have taken note that "plus-size" women actually *do* exercise, and are willing to spend their hard-earned dollars to do be comfortable and stylish while doing so. If you search online for "Plus Size Workout Clothing" you'll get page after page of results.

Be aware, however, that many of these places either have a limited selection of larger sizes in-store or only offer online sales. If you do need to purchase through a website, order in more than one size and color, so that you're saved the hassle of exchanging things through the mail. Returns are often free, but check the website policy just to be sure. Anyplace that has a brick-and-mortar store, such as Old Navy, will usually allow you to return your online purchases directly to the store. When you find a product line that seems to be made just for you, stock up!

Get a roundup of the best plus-size running gear, including size ranges, price ranges, shipping and return policies:

www.NotYourAverageRunner.com/
Gear-Guide

MATERIAL GIRL

Finding clothes that fit properly is more than half the battle, but fabric is extremely important too. As I mentioned above, cotton traps sweat, which can lead to a pretty miserable workout. The ideal material for running gear (including undies!) is a light, soft, synthetic blend that draws moisture away from your skin and dries quickly. Anything you wear on your bottom half will ideally have a lot of stretch to it as well. Avoid anything that's made mostly of cotton.

Most running clothes are now made from "moisture wicking" (also known as technical) fabrics which are designed to pull sweat away from your body to speed evaporation. The most important thing is that it be lightweight and dry quickly. If you pull your technical shirt out of the washing machine after the spin cycle and it feels almost dry, this is a good indicator that it will work well for you during a hot, sweaty run.

CARING FOR YOUR CLOTHES

Your running clothes (especially those sports bras) weren't cheap, so make the most of your money by caring for them properly. Always wash in cold water and never, ever put them in the dryer. Heat breaks down Spandex and Lycra, shortening their lifespan. Hang them on a rack when they come out of the washer and they'll be ready to wear in a few hours.

And when you're done with your workout, for Pete's sake, don't let your investment sit in a dark, closed hamper for days! Sweaty clothes are the perfect environment for bacteria to grow, and if you let them stew too long, they'll start to smell pretty ripe. At the very least, make sure to drop your clothes in an open basket, which will allow them to dry. And if you do find that your gear has an odor, soak it in a vinegar solution for a few hours and rewash.

PREVENTION OF CHAFING

Chafing is the bane of all runners, not just those that are overweight. Fortunately, there are many products to help you manage this uncomfortable problem. In addition to finding clothes that fit, look for shirts and tights with flat seams, and socks with minimal seams.

Bodyglide is an anti-chafing substance that looks a little like stick deodorant. Once applied, it feels completely dry, is invisible and odorless, and is resistant to sweat. Apply it anywhere seams irritate your skin, where you have skin-to-skin contact, or on those places on your feet that tend to rub against your shoes. You won't even know it's there, except when you undress after your run and realize you don't have angry red patches anywhere on your body! There are other products that have similar effects, but in my experience Bodyglide is the best. And definitely avoid Vaseline or any other petroleum jelly. Yes, it will reduce friction. It will also stain your clothes and feel sticky. Yuck!

Moleskin is an adhesive felt-like material that sticks to your skin and provides a barrier against friction. It is commonly used on the feet, but you can use it wherever you feel you need more protection than just Bodyglide. For example, when I use my iPhone armband, the edge of the strap rubs the inside of my arm raw. I place a small piece of moleskin right where the strap hits and Voila! Problem solved. It can be cut to any size and removes easily when your workout is done. If you're in a pinch and don't have any moleskin, a bandaid or athletic tape will work.

GADGETS AND OTHER FUN STUFF

What you choose to wear and bring with you on your run can help maintain your fitness mojo - or end up being a giant pain in the butt. For example, I used to tie my house key to my shoe laces, and then spend my entire run getting annoyed as it flopped around with every step. Nowadays, manufacturers are adding thoughtful details to their clothing lines, such as waistband key pockets, in an attempt to differentiate themselves from the pack. This is great news for you, because a functional garment can remove those pesky excuses for skipping a run, such as "I have no place to put my phone". When you're shopping, look for things like reflective strips, built-in pockets for a phone and extra-long sleeves with thumbholes to keep your hands warm in the winter. Or consider a lightweight wristband with a key/ID pocket. You can find them at most running stores, or look around on Pinterest to find instructions on making your own.

In addition to functional running gear, there are countless gadgets out there that allow you to gather data about your workouts. If you've got a smartphone with GPS, you can download an app (such as RunKeeper) that tracks how fast and far you ran, with the added bonus of calling out interval cues along the way. If you get lost, the GPS can lead you right back home..

If you don't want to carry a smartphone while you run, but still want the benefits of GPS, try a GPS watch that does all of the above while attached to your wrist. They are a bit bigger than a regular watch, but still lightweight enough that you won't notice it. After you run, stats are downloaded to your computer so you can review them with ease. The downside? Cost. Technology isn't cheap.

Don't care about GPS but still want to time your intervals? Go old school with a digital watch (such as the Timex Ironman), or pick up a simple, inexpensive and sweat-proof clip-on timer like the GymBoss.

Fitness trackers have come a long way in the past five years. For about $100, you can get a model that saves your step data electronically so you can track your activity over time with a web-based program and smartphone app.

Heart rate monitors are another popular tool with runners, because they give you a good understanding of how hard your cardio-respiratory system is working when you run. You can get a simple system for under $100, which includes a wrist unit so you can easily keep an eye on your heart rate while you're running.

One caveat to using all this cool gear: keep it simple. If it takes you a half-hour to get yourself ready to run, you've probably got too much going on (or else you're a master at delay tactics). Running toys should motivate you to get out the door, not get in the way. So if you find yourself fiddling around with all of your gadgets instead of actually running, try subtracting a few to see how it goes.

DEALING WITH INJURIES

Truly addicted runners love talking about two things: their stats, and their injuries. Although you might never torture your coworkers with every last detail about your weekend 5K, the sad truth is that at some point in the future, you're likely to experience a body issue that requires rest and healing. If you're lucky, your injuries will be mild and resolve quickly. Many of you will not be so fortunate, however, and you'll need to deal with the annoyance of taking a break from your beloved routine. This is the reality of any sport based on repetitive motion, but it doesn't mean you are doomed to failure.

In fifteen years of running I've had a lot of injuries. Achilles tendinitis, patellar tendinitis, plantar fasciitis, shin splints, bruised toes, IT band issues ... you name it, it seems like I've had it, and managed my way through it. The main lesson I've learned? Injuries heal if you let them. The problem is, taking the time to let them heal can be a big challenge.

Pain is your body's way of telling you it needs attention. Your body is smart! Listen to what it says, and learn the difference between discomfort, the voice of your inner mean girl and actual pain. You can run through discomfort and you should *always* ignore the negative voices in your head, but nine times out of ten you should not run through true pain.

When you think you're injured, or have a chronic pain that just won't go away, do your research. There are countless resources available online or in books. Ask other runners or stop by your local running store. Make an appointment with a specialist or physical therapist. The more you know, the more effective you can be in your recovery plan.

Forcing yourself to take a break, even if it's just for a week, is not always easy. You've just gotten yourself into a routine that you love and it feels amazing. You're afraid that if you lose your momentum you'll never get back on track. You feel angry, frustrated, and defeated. This is a chance for your mean girl to step up, telling you that your body has betrayed you, that you've failed yet again, and that you'll never be a real runner. The next thing you know, a week of rest has turned into three months of cupcake and wine-fueled pity parties–and you've proven all of those mean thoughts true. How do I know? Because I've been there. Many times.

To the negative mind, rest and quitting look a lot alike. They both involve not running, sometimes losing hard-won endurance and aerobic capacity, and perhaps even weight gain. But that's where the similarities end. Quitting is a result of giving up, negative thinking, and loss of confidence. Rest is a result of loving your body enough to care for it properly. If taking a break from running for a few weeks or months means the difference between full recovery, or causing further damage (and potentially not running ever again), the choice is clear. So if you want to be a runner for the next twenty-plus years, set yourself up for success by taking care of your body right now.

There's no need to panic about losing fitness during a rest break. Just because you can't run doesn't necessarily mean you can't exercise. Find another activity that doesn't aggravate your injury, such as walking, pool running, yoga, cycling, swimming, rowing–even the elliptical machine is better than nothing–to maintain a baseline fitness level. After you're cleared to start running again, I guarantee you will get back to your pre-injury levels of fitness, and that you will lose any weight you gained. It might not happen overnight, but there's no rush. You'll do it the same way you did the first time around: with consistency, patience and time. In the meantime, the rest might do your body a world of good, allowing everything to rejuvenate–not just the damaged parts.

And while you're resting? Stretch. A lot. You should always stretch after every workout, but it's even more important when you're taking a break to heal. Muscles can get extremely tight when they don't get much exercise, so spend a few minutes a day working on this aspect of your fitness and it will be much easier to get back into your groove when the time comes.

The reality is that you will probably get injured at some point. Expect it, take the time you need to heal and you'll come out stronger than before.

SAFETY GEAR

Unless all of your running is done on a treadmill, safety gear is something you need to understand. If you're running near traffic, you need make yourself as visible as possible to oncoming drivers. Wear bright clothes and/or a reflective vest, attach a blinking light to your shirt, choose garments with reflective strips–anything to draw attention to your presence on the side of the road. If you're running in a poorly lit area after dark, use a small headlamp to see where you're going. Finally, always carry ID with you, either a driver's license or an identifying wristband (such as RoadID) with your name, emergency contact, and medical alerts.

NUTRITION

Everyone's body is different, and there is no single nutritional plan that fits all. That being said, there are a few basic rules to follow to ensure your best performance:

- Feed yourself the highest quality fuel possible, at all times. This means avoiding processed foods, eating lots of produce, choosing high quality protein, sticking to complex carbs (rather than highly refined grains and sugar) and–yes, really–including some fat in your diet. I like to follow Michael Pollan's rule of thumb: If your great-grandmother wouldn't recognize it as food, don't eat it.

- A hydrated body performs better, so drink a fair amount of water each day. Unless you're running for two hours or more, or have a diagnosed electrolyte deficiency, you do not need to rehydrate with a sports drink. They are mostly just sugar. Stick to plain water, or add fruit for flavor.

- Avoid big meals in the couple hours before a run–if you're hungry, have a small snack such as a piece of fruit or a handful of nuts instead. Unless you're planning to run for more than an hour, your muscles should have enough stored fuel to get you through your workout on an empty stomach. Your body diverts blood flow away from non-essential organs when you're exercising, to make sure your muscles are properly supplied with oxygen. This includes your digestive track. That means any food that isn't easily absorbed will lie like a rock in your stomach while you run, because your body is busy doing other things. It is no fun to run with a bellyache. It's even less fun to stop running so you can puke.

- Consume alcohol in moderation, and never, ever, before a run, because it clouds your judgment and impairs your reflexes. Alcohol dehydrates your body and contains no real nutritive value (except for red wine, which I consider to be an essential food group). I prefer to avoid it completely for the couple days leading up to a big race or extra long run.

CONCLUSION

If you've made it this far, you're either over-the-moon excited to get busy with your new running addiction, or you're determined to get your money's worth. Either way, thanks for sticking with me to the end.

If I've done my job, I've convinced you that running will help you build up your self-esteem and make you feel like a rock star. Just beware–running is like a drug. If you use it regularly, you might get hooked. The addiction process has four stages:

1. Experimentation

Self-explanatory. At this point, running is just a way to mix up your workout routine, have a little fun, and find out what all the fuss is about. You might run a couple times a month, and it feels pretty good. What's the harm in experimenting, right?

2. Regular use

Now you're running a few times a week–because you really, reeeaaallly, like it. It's possible that you're hanging out with some new friends, people that spend a lot of time running, talking about running, and reading about running. You've begun to invest in running paraphernalia, and you're speaking the lingo: "Dude, I had such a great tempo run this weekend. It felt like I was flying!"

3. Risky use

It's getting all kinds of crazy up in here. You've rearranged your work schedule to make sure you can run at lunch, and curtail your drinking on nights before an early morning run. On Christmas morning, your family waits patiently to open presents while you get your run in, and one of your presents is a gift certificate for a running coach. Withdrawal symptoms appear when you have to skip a few days. Your old friends are starting to ask questions, and considering an intervention.

4. Dependency

At this point, you're beyond help. The addiction has infiltrated every aspect of your life. Your skin is glowing, self-confidence oozes from your pores, and you are actively recruiting others to your lifestyle.

Obviously, I'm in stage four.

In all seriousness, though, what I hope you've learned from our time together is that you absolutely *can* be a runner in the body you have right now. You are not too fat, your legs are not too short, and your fitness level is right where it needs to be. Runners come in all shapes, sizes, and abilities. There's room for everyone.

And since I'm terrible at goodbyes, I'm just going to leave you with a top ten list (in the grand traditions of both David Letterman and Moses). Call it the Ten Commandments of Running, if you like:

10. If you run, you are a runner.
9. Running is uncomfortable. Not impossible. You're capable of much more than you know.
8. It doesn't matter how many times you start over. Running will always be there for you.

7. Find your bliss. Understand why you run, or why you *want* to run. Make a list, keep adding to it over time, and refer to it regularly.

6. The back of the pack is a great place to be. Seriously.

5. Consistency, patience, and time get results. Your body will improve at its own pace, and if you stick with it, you'll get there. Don't rush it. Savor the journey.

4. If you fail to plan, you plan to fail. Expect the unexpected, and be ready.

3. Stop worrying about what everyone else thinks about you. Their opinion of you is not the problem–your opinion is the only one that counts. Start believing you are awesome, and you will be.

2. Find the good in every single run, even if it is as simple as saying "I ran today."
And finally,

1. Get out there and be an example of what is possible. You never know who you might inspire.

Stick to these guidelines, and you'll have many fabulous miles ahead of you.

To make the most of your running experience, grab one (or all!) of these free gifts from my website:

The Not Your Average Runner Manifesto:

www.NotYourAverageRunner.com/Manifesto

Plus-Size Running Gear Shopping Guide:

www.NotYourAverageRunner.com/Gear-Guide

Beginner's Guide

www.NotYourAverageRunner.com/start

Ready to take it to the next level?

Join the Virtual Running Club!

www.NotYourAverageRunner.com/jointhecommunity

GRATITUDE

This book could not have happened without the help, wisdom, love and kindness of the many fabulous people in my life! I am humbled and grateful beyond measure by your unwavering support.

To my parents: Thank you for loving me and teaching me that I can do or be anything I want. I wish you were here to see what you set in motion.

To Martha, Tom, Kerry and Paul: You are the best siblings a girl could hope for. Thank you for always being there with a kind word and for believing in me. It means more than you could ever know.

To Abby, Amanda, Gina, McKenzie and Nina: Thank you for sharing your own personal thoughts on running, and for allowing me to put them out there in the world. Your words will help so many others. They most certainly helped me.

To all my girlfriends and girl-boss-friends: Thank you for listening, supporting, inspiring and never, EVER doubting me (and for calling me out on my shenanigans).

To Angela Lauria and the Author Incubator team: Thank you for bringing this book from dream to reality. I could not have done this without you. You have changed my life.

To Brooke Castillo: I have no words to express the deep gratitude I feel to have worked and studied with you. I am forever changed for the better.

To *ALL* of my family, friends and clients, both near and far: Thank you for the never-ending encouragement. Thank you for the emails, for listening, for talking it out, for reading my work, for sharing it with everyone you know, and for sending your positive energy my way. There have been times over the past few months when I've struggled with writing, with training for a half-marathon, or just generally questioned my life path. At those moments, I often hear a quiet voice in my head telling me to keep going. I know these voices are coming from all of you. It is amazing to have such a fabulous support system.

To the Morgan James Publishing team: Special thanks to David Hancock, CEO & Founder for believing in me and my message. To my Author Relations Manager, Tiffany Gibson, thanks for making the process seamless and easy. Many more thanks to everyone else, but especially Jim Howard, Bethany Marshall, and Nickcole Watkins.

To every single stranger that has ever cheered me on during a race, or shouted 'keep up the good work' when they see me chugging along, THANK YOU.

To my own body - legs, heart, lungs and all the rest - you rock. Thank you for not giving up.

ABOUT THE AUTHOR

Jill Angie is a running coach and personal trainer who wants to live in a world where everyone is free to feel fit and fabulous at any size. She started the Not Your Average Runner movement in 2013 to show that runners come in all shapes, sizes and speeds, and since then has assembled 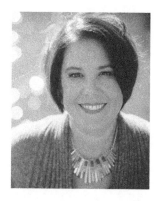 a global community of revolutionaries that are taking the running world by storm. If you would like to be part of the movement, visit www.NotYourAverageRunner.com to find out more!

THANK YOU

Thank you for reading this book. It was a true labor of love, and if it affected you in some way, I invite you to share your thoughts by writing a review on Amazon or Facebook!

CONTACT INFO/SOCIAL MEDIA

Jill@NotYourAverageRunner.com
www.NotYourAverageRunner.com
Facebook.com/NotYourAverageRunner
Instagram.com/NotYourAverageRunner

Free Chapter from
Not Your Average 5K

Hey there! If you picked up this book, I'm assuming you have a desire, somewhere deep down in your soul, to do a 5K someday—or else you're stuck on a 13 hour flight to Australia with nothing else to do and you've read every other book on your Kindle. Either way, I'm glad you're here!

Not Your Average 5K is a sequel to my first book, *Not Your Average Runner: Why You're Not Too Fat to Run, and the Skinny on How to Start Today*, but you don't need to have read it to get the most out of this book. Of course, it's a pretty awesome book—both hilarious and educational—so feel free to download it right now, wink wink.

OK, ready to go? Great! First of all, I have great news for you.

This book is going to rock your world.

Throughout the rest of this book, I'm going to give you everything you need to start and finish your first 5K. You'll get an awesome training program, figure out how to fit running into your packed schedule, learn how to run with proper form and breathing, stay motivated even when you're tired or busy, and fuel your body like a real runner (and I don't mean eating nothing but carrots and protein shakes!). Most importantly, you're going to triumphantly cross that finish line like an absolute rock star.

You're going to get there in just 2 months, too. How are we going to do it? Well, we're going to follow a tried and tested system that I've created called YOUR FIRST 5K. Each letter corresponds to a week in your training program, and has a very specific purpose:

Y. **Why** do a 5K?
O. **Orient** yourself for success
U. **Understand** the basics
R. **Resourceful** running
F. **Fuel** properly
I. **Initiate** yourself into the club

R. Resiliant Running

S. Stay motivated when life gets in the way

T. Try it out—race day rehearsal and strategies for success

5K.5K week, time to put everything together and race!

You'll have a homework assignment for each chapter, as well as three training runs to complete each week. The program is designed to properly build up your strength and endurance so you can show up on race day ready to run and have a blast.

If you're thinking "But I've already done a 5K, this isn't the book for me," I have good news. You can still get a lot out of this book! It's not just for brand-new beginners, and even if you've got a few under your belt already, I guarantee you'll learn something new.

Before we jump in, however, I need you to do a few things. First, make sure you read the entire book before you officially start the training plan. I know you're excited to get started, but I promise that taking a few hours to read everything from start to finish will give you the best chance of success. It's short. Draw a scented bubble bath, pour a glass of wine, and carve out the next couple of hours just for you. Or hide out in your car with a latte while the kids are at soccer practice. It's all good. You're officially on your way to your first 5K and that's all that matters.

After you're done reading, download and print your training plan. This will be your guide for everything you do throughout the rest of this book[1].

Finally–and this might be the most important step of all–pick out a reward for yourself for hitting your goal! It can be anything at all—as simple as treating yourself to a celebratory meal with your family, or a super deluxe payoff like getting a new kitchen (like one of my clients did, and she still hasn't invited me over for dinner!). Whatever you choose, make sure it is meaningful to you, because you'll use it to help boost your motivation throughout the process. Write it down on a post-it note and stick it on your fridge. And here's an idea: take a picture of your note and email it to me at reward@NotYourAverageRunner.com—and I'll check back with you in two months to see if you've earned it yet!

Who is this book for?

This book is for anyone (and I mean AN-Y-ONE) who wants to complete their first 5K. That means you don't even have to be a runner right now. As long as you can walk for 3 miles, you will be able to do a 5K in two months. I promise.

1

Also, this book is designed to train you to finish that 5K in a way that feels good to you, both mentally and physically. That means you can walk, run, skip, or even disco dance your way across the finish line. Now, if you've already done a 5K (or two… or five), this doesn't mean you won't get anything out of this book. Just the opposite, in fact. There is a truckload of helpful information here that will help you take your 5K performance to the next level.

Not convinced yet? OK, fine. Let me introduce you to a couple of my favorite people.

Meet Cindy.

Cindy just turned 46, has a 9-year old son, and weighs about 75 pounds more than she'd like to. She's stopped and started a ton of fitness programs in the past–always with the best of intentions–but each and every time she loses interest after a couple of weeks and now her bedroom closet has a shameful pile of yoga mats, kettle bells and fitness bands gathering dust. Every time her husband complains about it, she's all, "Oh, I'm going to start using those next week!" but another month comes and goes and soon there's another fitness gadget added to the pile.

She knows her husband loves her and supports her, but she's totally lost her sexy spark and feels old and frumpy. She used to love to get dressed up to go out, but lately she'd rather stay on the couch with her family and a big pile of take-out food. She's just too tired all the time to do anything else.

Still, she does go for a walk around the neighborhood a few times a month, and even throws in an occasional jogging interval when she thinks nobody is looking. In fact, one time she ran for a minute straight and felt like such a rock star. That night, she dreamed about running effortlessly like a Kenyan. It was amazing.

The next morning she woke up and told her husband and he laughed his butt off.

"You? Running? Um, I hate to break it to you honey, but your track record for exercise is pretty bad. You're just not the type of person that likes to move."

Grrrr. Sometimes she thinks that doing a 5K would be the best revenge, if for no other reason than to prove other people wrong.

Then her son chipped in:

"Yeah Mom, the last time we went on vacation you just sat and read a book while everyone else went for a bike ride. But that's OK, if you got all skinny I wouldn't be able to use your tummy as a pillow when we're watching TV."

Ooof. That one really hurt.

The truth is, Cindy does enjoy her occasional walks and believes she could do a 5K or even a longer distance. Her problem is that she stalls out every time she thinks about all that's involved. Making time in her busy schedule. Finding cute running clothes that fit and don't make her look like an elephant. Learning how to breathe properly. Getting the courage to actually sign up for a race. It's flat-out overwhelming and keeps her on the couch.

But she knows that if she sets a goal and goes public with it, she's less likely to back out. After giving it some thought, Cindy picks a small, local 5K about 2 months away and signs up. She marks it on her calendar and (gulp) tells her family. They laugh and say they'll believe it when they see it.

"Game on!" Cindy thinks.

Cindy's challenges will be reprogramming her established habits by creating new ones. She will also have to manage her beliefs that her husband and son see her as a quitter. The good news is that once Cindy begins to see herself as someone who follows through on her commitments, her family will be able to view her that way too. She will need to remember that running will feel hard at first, but that doesn't mean she's not good at it—the longer she sticks with it, the easier it will get.

Now meet Sarah.

Sarah is 37, with two daughters aged ten and four. She's got an amazing career and gets promoted year after year, and always gets complimented on how competent and confident she is at work. And she's making a ton of money, which means her family can have a gorgeous home and take some really fabulous vacations. From the outside, she has a dream life.

But inside, she feels like a total failure. She's struggled with body image for most of her life, and despite losing 124 pounds three years ago (and hitting her goal weight in just 18 months!) she still hates what she sees when she looks in the mirror. This is a huge disappointment because Sarah really believed that losing weight would make everything perfect.

To top it all off, she has to stay pretty active to maintain her weight loss. Spin class on Saturday mornings, elliptical and a few weight machines before work on Tuesdays and Thursdays, and most nights she walks for 30 minutes on the treadmill in her bedroom, which is when she catches up on her Netflix queue. She's getting pretty good at it too–she can knock out a little over two miles during that time.

Her sister keeps telling her she should start running, but *seriously*?! Sure, she works out a lot, but she's no athlete. Sarah's butt still wobbles and she will never get rid of all that loose skin on her belly and arms without surgery. Wearing a skimpy little tank top–or worse, just a sports bra (which is what runners wear, right?)–is out of the question. Runners are teeny tiny women with perfect bodies and flat stomachs. There's no way she'll ever be a runner. She just doesn't fit in.

Then one day her 9-year old asked to sign up for Girls on the Run during the next school year.

Crap.

This would be an awesome program for her daughter to join, because it not only teaches girls how to run, it also gives them life skills and confidence and teaches them to feel good about themselves.

But if her girls start running, won't they need a training partner? And shouldn't that be her?

Suddenly, Sarah is motivated to at least give it a try, because this is a great opportunity to spend time with her daughter and talk about body image and self-confidence. She's a little worried about keeping up, but she'll do anything to make her kids happy. So she gets her oldest registered for the program the next day, and shifts her schedule around so she can run while her daughter is at practice twice a week. Afterwards, they will chat about their progress in the car on the way home.

Like Cindy, Sarah will also have to manage her beliefs about herself. Despite being successful at weight loss and already a regular exerciser, Sarah does not see herself as an athlete because–in her opinion–she doesn't look like one. To get past this, Sarah will need to believe that athletes come in all shapes and sizes and that the appearance of her body has nothing to do with her fitness level. This will have a huge impact on her daughters too—because when they see their mom feeling confident, they'll naturally follow along.

Both Cindy and Sarah are very typical stories of someone who is not your average runner: someone who wasn't a "skinny mini" in high school, and for whom physical activity does not come easily. The good news is both of these amazing women went on to train for and complete their first 5K, had a ton of fun doing it, and even continued running afterwards. And you can too!

If you're still not quite sure, let me tell you a little about myself.

I'm 48, and I've been a runner, off and on, since 1998. During that time, my weight has fluctuated between 180 and 280 pounds–more than once– but it has never impacted my ability to train for and complete dozens of races, from 5K's to half marathons to triathlons.

When I first started running, a 5K wasn't even on my radar. I just wanted to lose weight, and decided to run laps around my block. Since I couldn't go more than 30 seconds at a time, that's exactly where I started. I would sprint for 30 seconds, completely out of breath, and walk for a minute or two to recover, over and over again until I'd completed four laps (two miles). Back then, most people didn't know about the run/walk interval method, they just kept adding a few minutes to their workout until they were running the entire time (or they gave up, because that's a *really* hard way to train for a 5K). As you'd expect, I got plenty of raised eyebrows and funny looks from my neighbors, all of them wondering why I was running like I was being chased by a bear and then suddenly stopping to walk.

This was in the middle of one of the hottest summers on record in eastern PA, and almost every run was difficult and uncomfortable. Most of the time, I thought I was going to pass out from the heat. At the time, cute workout clothes never came in anything larger than a size L, so I ran in long, thick cotton leggings, stretched so tightly I was always waiting for them to rip, and covered up the rest of my body in enormous men's cotton t-shirts that hung to my knees.

Needless to say, I sweated my butt off that summer, but eventually I got stronger, running a couple of minutes at a time, and learned how to pace myself so that I was jogging at a comfortable pace instead of racing around like a lunatic. It even started to feel good, and I began to realize that my life in general felt so much easier when I ran regularly.

Then someone told me about a local 5K. I had no idea such a thing existed, but it sounded like fun so I signed up and started training in earnest.

Race day came, and I lined up to start with 100 others who looked like real athletes–thin, fit, and wearing actual running clothes. I felt totally out of place. When the starting gun went off, I quickly found myself at the back of the pack.

There was a choice to be made: I could feel bad about being left in the dust and suffer for the entire event, or I could run at my own speed without stressing out, giving it my best effort while having fun. I chose the latter, and finished in 42 minutes. Because there were only 100 runners, I was almost dead last. But it was one of the proudest moments of my life because that was the moment I knew I was a runner.

It was so powerful that years later I still get teary thinking about how it felt to cross that finish line. I want you to have that feeling too.

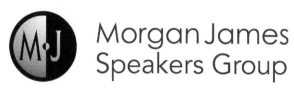

Morgan James
Speakers Group

www.TheMorganJamesSpeakersGroup.com

We connect Morgan James published
authors with live and online events
and audiences who will benefit
from their expertise.

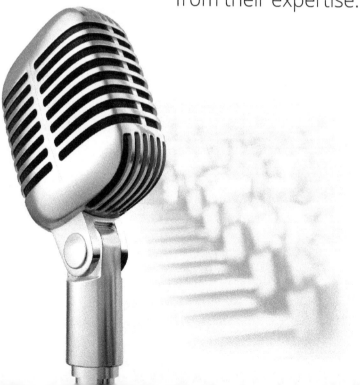